Insulin Resistance Solution

Prevent diabetes, restore metabolism, eliminate abdominal fat and stay fit - with many unique recipes

Antony Jason Willfour
PAGEMAN PUBLISHERS

Lack of
Quality Sleep

Excess Carbs
Consumption

Lack of
Exercise

Chronic Illness
& Inflammation

Abdominal Fat
& Obesity

Genetic
Susceptibility

Insulin
Resistance

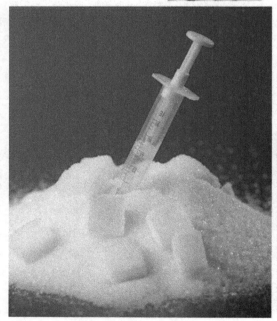

prevent loss of

with non-conducting

insuli

which regulates gl

in the blood.

Table of Contents

Introduction

Insulin resistance is one of the most widespread health problems affecting western culture.

It affects at least 86 million adults in the USA alone[1], and it's estimated that 80% of overweight people suffer from insulin resistance...

Insulin resistance is one of the most insidious health problems out there – once it develops it can be difficult to spot the symptoms, but it will wreck your energy levels and ruin your efforts live a healthy and happy life, making it harder for you to lose weight and gain muscle.

But many people don't know what it is, let alone realize they have it!

Unable to Lose Weight?

...Insulin resistance makes it easier to *gain* fat but harder to *lose* it.

Finding it Difficult to Build Muscle Tone?

...Insulin resistance makes it more difficult for your body to build and maintain muscles.

Do You Feel Often Feel, Tired and Hungry?

...Insulin resistance causes you to feel fatigued and creates cravings for junk food.

But there's good news too...

You can reverse insulin resistance *without* drugs *or* surgery. A little knowledge and education combined with the right diet and lifestyle changes can help you to heal your body and feel better than ever before.

Inside you'll learn:

- Exactly how Insulin resistance develops in the body

- Signs you may be suffering from insulin resistance

- How Insulin resistance could be affecting your health, weight and energy levels

- The best route for overcoming insulin resistance

- The insulin resistance diet, including my favorite insulin resistance beating recipes

- Top tips and strategies for reducing insulin resistance and becoming healthier

PART 1: UNDERSTANDING INSULIN RESISTANCE

What exactly is Insulin?

Insulin is not very well understood by most people. You may know that it has something to do with diabetes and a lot of people with diabetes have to inject themselves with insulin... but for many people that is the extent of our understanding.

Insulin is neither entirely good nor bad; it is a hormone that is vital to our health, but in the wrong amounts can also be deadly. It is life-saving for those with type 1 diabetes but can speed up the progress to type 2 diabetes and obesity for those with poor diets.

Insulin is the body's way of regulating glucose in the bloodstream, which when excess in toxic amounts, sends it to the only other two other places the body where it can be stored – the liver or the muscles. Although glucose is one of the main sources of energy for the human body (from the breakdown of all carbohydrates and sugars – think bread, potatoes, sugar etc), the human body can only store a finite amount of glucose.

Insulin is produced by the beta cells of the pancreas in response to ingested sugar, even some sugar substitutes can activate a small insulin response. The insulin flows through the blood stream and links with cells and unlocks them, allowing those cells to absorb glucose for immediate use or to make their own stores of longer lasting glycogen. It also allows cells to better absorb amino acids, the building blocks of proteins and muscle. Insulin prompts the liver to store glycogen and if there is any extra from there it gets converted into body fat (note: dietary *sugar* is converted to body fat in this process, not dietary fat. We'll return to this later).

An absence of insulin has the opposite effect; the liver breaks down glycogen into glucose and excretes it for the body to use because it does not have glucose in the diet and body fat is metabolized.

Insulin is a very old evolutionary trick which allows animals to survive periods of starvation followed by satiation and avoid the damaging effects of glucose in the blood stream. As prehistoric humans, we largely ate meat and fibrous plants, which broke down slowly to release glucose over time. When we could get some berries or honey our bodies saw huge glucose spikes. Though all of this glucose was of a high quality energy, glucose has a corrosive effect when in the blood stream. To avoid this damage, insulin was released by the pancreas to immediately get that glucose where it needed to be, (the muscles), and stored the rest in the liver and body fat to prepare for when the body couldn't get anything to eat.

Prehistoric humans didn't need insulin spikes too often, but when we did, it allowed us to use that high quality energy and also allowed us to store the excess as fat and liver stores of glycogen. So, when we found a berry patch during the stone age it was not inherently unhealthy to eat only berries for the whole day because chances were that we were not going to find such a berry bush for a while, perhaps for the whole winter – frequent periods of fasting and starvation were part of the nature of life for our ancestors. **Problems start when we find that "berry patch" every day,** and we never go through periods of real physiological starvation. What was designed as a quick response system to the occasional sugar rush became used several times a day.

Insulin Resistance

Glucose is the preferred immediate source of energy for our muscles, brain and countless other specialized cells. Any carbohydrate can be broken down within a certain amount of time to create more glucose, but since glucose is corrosive when in the blood it gets converted and stored in the cells as a denser collection of glucose known as glycogen. Our muscles will use any readily available glucose first and then use its stores of glycogen. When insulin comes around to distribute glucose, our cells use that energy, but also take enough glucose to replenish their stores of glycogen.

Insulin's rather elegant system for storing toxic glucose in the muscle and liver doesn't function so well when the body is frequently exposed to high levels of blood glucose.

Frequent or prolonged spikes in blood glucose can cause the body's cells to become resistant to insulin. If our blood sugar and insulin spike when our glycogen stores are mostly full and our cell's energy requirements are low then the cell will not be receptive to any insulin because it doesn't need glucose. This leads to a resistance to insulin as the connections normally used to accept it begin changing and it becomes difficult for cells to accept insulin, even if they really needed glucose.

Imagine insulin as a door-to-door Girl Scout selling cookies (glucose). When we first see those girl scouts we are craving

10

cookies and we (muscle/liver cells) order as many as we can eat (glucose) and store (glycogen) and everything is fantastic. Now imagine you get your cookies and another girl scout comes to sell cookies. Well, you're fully stocked on cookies, so maybe you buy just one box. Then, a day after that, another girl scout comes and you just have to turn her away. Now, the poor girl scouts have too many cookies left to sell and they might get their sisters or parents (more insulin) to take some boxes around the neighborhood (high blood sugar) until they finally sell. In a sense, this is how insulin resistance begins, but it gets much worse from here.

As we mentioned before, **repeated levels of high insulin secretion were not normal for our prehistoric ancestors**. The intended role of insulin in the body was to signal the muscles and other cells to fill up their depleted stores of glycogen and use the glucose available. When insulin was released, the cells usually *needed* that glucose and gladly opened up to receive the glucose. If we fill those stores and don't use them, then when insulin comes to deliver some glucose those cells can't take in any more glucose and become *resistant* to insulin. The number of insulin receptor sites on the surface of the cells decrease in number as does their efficiency.

Blood glucose is increased as it has nowhere to go and the pancreas just sees that the levels of glucose in the blood are still too high and produces more insulin. What results is too much corrosive glucose persisting in the bloodstream as well as an excess of insulin, which can cause problems of its own.

In a modern carbohydrate focused diet only serious endurance athletes can consistently deplete their glycogen stores to prevent this resistance. Even those who exercise still tend to overload their cells with glucose on a daily basis.

So, it might seem easy to just deplete those glycogen stores and you can eat more sugar, but it is not that simple. As cells repeatedly turn away insulin, they become used to doing that and begin to be less receptive to insulin even when they need glucose. So, even when cells need glucose they begin to need far more insulin than normal to be able to accept it causing insulin levels to routinely rise far more than a dose of carbohydrates should need.

Too much insulin can cause some problems, especially when cells become resistant. Insulin will convert glucose to visceral fat as a last option. This fat surrounds the internal organs at first, and then grows around the abdomen. As fat grows by adipose cells accepting and converting glucose into fat, they can also reach a point where they have a difficult time accepting any more and become insulin

> **Early Stages on Insulin Resistance**
>
> 1. The level of blood glucose stays higher longer because glucose can't be stored in the muscle and liver. Getting toxic glucose out of the bloods stream is one of insulin's main jobs and periods of elevated blood sugar are bad news — causing inflammation and forming advanced glycated end products (AGEs) that cause aging.
> 2. The pancreas increases insulin production to compensate for the insulin resistance of the cells in the muscle and liver. Even insulin can be toxic in high levels and permanently insulated insulin levels cause other problems like···
>
>   a. Having a harder time burning stored fat because of this increased level of insulin. Fat burning occurs in the absence of insulin so elevated insulin levels stop this process happening.

resistant themselves. With nowhere to go, the glucose usually ends up being converted to LDL cholesterol and wanders the blood, clogging arteries.

As you can see, insulin resistance can lead to an increase in both our blood glucose and insulin levels, both of which have negative health consequences, but physical health can be affected – **fat is easily accumulated and hard to lose, whereas muscle is difficult to gain and easy to lose.**

13

You can see that insulin resistance can be a serious business, both for the state of our long-term health and our physical health and self-esteem. What are some signs of insulin resistance?

There are many symptoms of insulin resistance and excess insulin production known as hyperinsulinemia. One of the more obvious symptoms is high blood sugar, which can persist for much longer than normal. Fatigue and sleepiness are also quite common as it becomes difficult for the body to regulate its own energy. Feeling tired after sleeping for 9 hours is normal because your body can't quite get glucose to the muscles and brain to help wake you up. The way glucose, insulin and insulin resistance affect the brain are quite complex and are still being extensively studied, but we know that some people will have problems getting adequate energy to the brain. This can cause periods of brain fogginess as well as difficulty focusing. There are also links to the development of depression. Insulin also inhibits the excretion of excess sodium through the kidneys and therefore causes excess sodium, which causes high blood pressure and increases the risk of heart disease and stroke.

Insulin works in several ways to increase body fat. Insulin actually stimulates the appetite causing you to crave more even as your body struggles to deal with the excess glucose it already has. We know that insulin will turn glucose into fat and store it around the organs and waist after supplying the necessary cells, but with insulin resistance, more insulin is produced so turning sugar into fat happens almost automatically because the liver and muscles become insulin resistant before the fat cells do. More insulin is released for smaller amounts of sugars, but the insulin resistance in the liver and muscles causes a much higher percentage of glucose to be turned into fat rather than being made available as ready fuel.

Insulin resistance also causes inflammation throughout the body and puts strain on multiple organs. The sugars in the blood corrode blood vessels and the kidneys have the job of getting rid of the excess glucose in the blood. As the glucose filters through, it can damage the kidneys and combined with the extra sodium retention, can cause the formation of painful kidney stones. The kidneys require a great deal of water to excrete the extra sugar so it is not uncommon to be dehydrated and thirsty. Repetitive high blood sugars can also cause cirrhosis, or scarring, on the liver **similar to the scarring seen on the livers of alcoholics**. Whole body inflammation caused by the abundance of blood sugar has several of its own symptoms including chronic muscle and joint pain, irritable bowel syndrome and rashes and red and irritated eyes. Chronic inflammation is also linked with some of the biggest killers in the modern world including heart disease, stroke and cancer.

Although these symptoms might sound very serious and sobering, it's important to realize that the initial stages of insulin resistance may develop and go unnoticed. You may not present any symptoms initially and any that do appear may be difficult to detect.

You might be thinking you're in the clear because you rarely feel fatigued, perform well at work or you're confident that you exercise enough and you're not overweight. However, the reality is that everyone's body is very different and we all respond to sugar, insulin and even inflammation quite differently. The brain responds differently to a variety of factors, so you may not have symptoms like brain fogginess, or perhaps you just power through when you're thinking becomes sluggish or you just assume your occasional brain fog is normal and happens to everyone.

 You may have rashes caused by chronic inflammation, but those could be mistaken for any number of harmless rashes. You might have fatigue, but you just convince yourself that you are naturally a bit lazy. You could be overweight, but you might think it's those fatty burgers and not that sugary breakfast cereal. You could even have several damaging internal symptoms without realizing it. If you have repetitive kidney damage it can be very difficult to realize it and if you are young it might take a lot of damage and build up before painful kidney stones develop.

The Questions you need to ask yourself to determine whether insulin resistance could be a problem for you are: frequently consuming high carbohydrate and/or sugary food? Do you experience any of the following symptoms:

- Brain fogginess and inability to focus

- Intestinal bloating

- Sleepiness, especially after meals

- Weight gain, fat storage, difficulty losing weight – particularly around the abdomen

- Increased blood pressure

- Depression

- Increased hunger

- Acanthosis nigricans (skin condition)[2]

Also remember that black, Hispanic, Asian and American Indian groups are more at risk as well as those aged 40+ [3]·[4].

Just because you don't know you have insulin resistance doesn't mean that you aren't damaging your body and if you don't do anything about it serious life-threatening complications can occur.

Consequences of Untreated Insulin Resistance

You know some of the symptoms of insulin resistance, but what happens if nothing is done and the trend continues? One of the most troubling results is that you begin to lack energy, because your cells are so resistant to receiving new glucose. When your body is exhausted it craves more high-energy carbohydrates. This is a vicious cycle, which quickly worsens insulin resistance already present.

Another contributing factor is the accumulation of body fat. Too much body fat lessens the impact of the hormone leptin, which causes any feelings of fullness to be fleeting, further increasing your hunger. The less sugar that is able to get to your cells, the quicker your body will turn to breaking down your own muscles for fuel which means you will have less muscle mass to burn off sugars and you will become weaker and even less likely to exercise. As a double whammy, insulin also opens muscle cells to absorb amino acids for muscle growth; insulin resistance means that those building blocks can't gain access either; so your muscles break down while being denied the materials to build them back up again, making it extremely difficult to build and maintain muscle mass.

Insulin resistance can severely damage your organs as well. We talked about scarring of the liver and kidney stones but those are just precursors to more serious problems. The kidneys and liver filter out the toxins from the blood and the liver also creates, converts and stores energy and hormones. Damage to the kidney causes swelling as fluid builds up throughout the body, and continued damage can lead to painful or bloody urination. The kidneys release hormones related to red blood cell creation and kidney damage can create decreased red blood cells causing anemia.

Liver damage can cause similar symptoms and can cause a chronic dull pain in the abdomen, itchy skin and nausea. The liver also creates hormones which interact with your thyroid and a damaged liver can send too much or too little of the necessary hormones throwing the thyroid out of balance. Thyroid problems vary greatly, but can include symptoms such as muscle weakness, heart palpitations and lethargy.

Lastly, the extreme conclusion is that chronic insulin resistance can lead to diabetes. We have talked about how damaging high blood sugar can be, but we haven't mentioned the damage that's done to the organ trying to regulate the blood sugar; the pancreas. The pancreas produces insulin in its beta cells. A fully functioning pancreas can produce a huge amount of insulin, but the problem is that glucose actually damages these beta cells as they are working to produce more insulin. As mentioned before, insulin resistance causes more and more insulin to be produced, but progressive insulin resistance means progressive damage to the beta cells. It's like a factory getting more and more orders while simultaneously getting downsized. After a while, it is too damaged to keep up and instead of producing far more insulin than normal for a comparative amount of glucose, it produces much less. Once this happens it's classified as type 2 diabetes and blood sugar can no longer be effectively managed by the body. Now even if your cells are ready to accept sugar, your body cannot produce enough insulin on its own to get glucose to all the cells that need it.

Late Stages on Insulin Resistance

1. When the liver becomes insulin resistant, it's unable convert thyroid hormone T4 into hormone T3, leading to thyroid problems, furthering slowing the metabolism and exacerbating the condition.

2. The excess sugar can destroy nerve tissue leading to nerve damage and pain in the extremities, and retinopathy can develop, leading to loss of eyesight.

3. Eventually the damaged pancreas loses the ability to produce insulin, leading to insulin-dependent, Type 2 diabetes.

We will discuss the non-dietary factors you can use to combat insulin resistance, but the biggest factor for insulin resistance is your diet. People are quick to dismiss their diet because it is an automatic part of their day, an afterthought. People also have a terribly hard time when they are asked to change what they eat, especially when they are asked to give up sweets. Sweets and carbohydrates in general are the single biggest factor to developing insulin resistance. Glucose of any amount triggers insulin production, and we know that even a bit of insulin resistance can prompt a vicious cycle of worsening resistance.

The first step in treating insulin resistance is normalizing insulin levels, which mean reducing consumption of carbohydrates and sugary foods.

This means reduction in foods like bread, potatoes, white rice, noodles, pasta and sugary foods like sweets, candy, sugared cereal etc. One of the key factors to examine when eating carbohydrates is the food's glycemic index, among many other nutritional factors. Glycemic index is a measure of how much a given food elevates your blood sugar an hour after consumption with 0 being none and 100 being pure glucose. While simple carb foods like doughnuts come in pretty high at 76 it can be surprising that foods like bagels, French fries, shredded wheat and even pizza all average in in the 70's on the glycemic index scale. Even some brands of whole wheat bread can have indexes of 70 or 80. When a healthy body is overwhelmed by sugar, it rushes out more insulin to handle it, causing resistance as the body's cells quickly fill up their stores of glycogen. We'll aim to cut out high glycemic carbs and sugars and replace them with low glycemic foods like meat, fish, vegetables, fruit, cheese and beans.

A current recommendation for diabetics and even those with insulin resistance is increased consumption of complex carbohydrates. The term complex carbohydrate is somewhat nebulous, referring generally to carbohydrate rich food with some fiber content, which slows their digestion, like brown bread. While complex carbohydrates are better than simple sugars that cause quick blood sugar spikes, simply switching your white bread for brown bread won't be enough to fight insulin resistance. Carbohydrates, simple or complex, will break down to glucose and will provoke insulin secretion. Whilst the slower sugar release from complex carbohydrates like brown pasta, rice and bread are better than their white counterparts, switching to naturally low GI foods like vegetables and beans will be more effective and provide a wider range of vitamins and nutrients to support the body during it's time of healing. If you feel that you are already struggling with insulin resistance it is best to minimise carbohydrates, even complex ones. The bottom line with insulin resistance and diabetes is that the body is no longer able to effectively process sugar, so any sugars can do more harm than good.

Energy Sources

You might be wondering where the body gets it energy from if carbohydrates are restricted, or worrying that lack of dietary sugars will lead to low energy or feelings of tiredness. The answer is that the body has systems for regulating blood sugar within certain limits. When our blood sugar drops the body will stabilize it by increasing the proportion of energy utilized from fatty acids.

The brain has a certain energy requirement for glucose, and the body gets round this by creating another type of substance for the brain to use during times of low blood sugar called ketones. The liver uses fatty acids to produce ketones during times of low blood sugar as energy for the brain and some other cells. You may have heard the term 'ketogenesis' or 'ketogenic diet' in regard to low carbohydrate diets — and it's this process to which the terms relate.

That being said, complex carbohydrates really are the better carbohydrate to eat if you don't already have insulin resistance because your body can handle the slow release of sugar more easily. To prevent the initial onset of insulin resistance, it is important to pace and limit your sugars.

If you do eat carbohydrates, try to make them nutrient dense and low glycemic index foods. Gluten free carbs such as quinoa can be a good carb to use while working to cut down on worse carbs as it has a good balance of minerals, protein and fiber while usually being around 50 or lower on the glycemic index. Many beans also have low GIs and can be a great choice.

Fruits can seem like a bad choice as some like watermelon have a GI of 70 but unless you eat dried fruit you are getting a lot of fiber as well as a lot of water which does a lot to balance out the amount of sugar you eat as well as the impact it has. Vegetables also have a great amount of fiber, vitamins and minerals in addition to their complex carbohydrates.

Outside of carbohydrate control, there are other foods that have a big impact on how your body processes sugar. Having a healthy balance of the right fats is important. Trans fats and diets full of processed oils and margarines can cause inflammation in the body and worsen the symptoms of insulin resistance. Healthy fats such as omega 3 fatty acids can improve insulin sensitivity, having the opposite effect of insulin resistance. Foods like the avocado provide an abundance of healthy fats and when eaten along with carbohydrates the healthy fats slow digestion and lessen the overall glycemic impact of a meal.

There are certain other foods that are excellent at fighting or reversing insulin resistance.

- The previously mentioned avocado not only has healthy fats, it also is full of fiber, which also slows digestion, makes you feel fuller longer and improves digestive health. It also provides plenty of B vitamins and potassium while being low in overall sugar.

- Cinnamon, in addition to being high in fiber, has amazing blood sugar regulation properties. Cinnamon slows digestion, which can lessen the impact of sugars, but it also binds with sugars and can manage blood sugar about as well as several common diabetes drugs.

- Eggs, yes the whole egg yolk and all, are amazing foods to ward of insulin resistance. They also have plenty of protein and healthy fats and also keep you very full for a long time and keep you from snacking on junk food.

- If you are not sensitive to it than most dairy is excellent as it balances moderate sugars with healthy fats and quality protein while providing a variety of vitamins and minerals. Go ahead a drink a glass of 2% or even whole milk or a bowl of Greek yoghurt and see how full you are, you might be surprised how long dairy can ward off sugar cravings.

- Sweet potatoes have a misleading name. Certainly they will raise your blood sugar right? Well, the complexity of sweet potatoes means that you can get different results by how it's prepared. It is possible to get a sweet tasting sweet potato dish with a GI of under 50 while also providing plenty of fiber and minerals.

- For those who are suffering from insulin resistance it is a good idea to get anti-inflammatory foods into the diet. Foods such as ginger and peppers simply lower inflammation with specific compounds while foods such as nuts and leafy vegetables lower inflammation by providing healthy fats and vitamin E.

Non-Dietary Factors of Insulin Resistance

Now, we know that you are what you eat, but there are other factors that determine if you can get insulin resistance and how well you can fight it off and prevent diabetes. We know that insulin resistance begins because cells (mainly muscle cells) are full up on their glycogen stores and become less responsive to insulin because of that. Well if you don't let your cells keep full stores for very long than you are much less likely to start any kind of insulin resistance. If you haven't yet figured it out, the answer is regular exercise.

When you exercise, you burn up fuel and when your muscles burn up the glucose that is ready to go to the cells, they then burn up available glucose in the blood and then break down their stores of glycogen. So, when you exercise, you burn up any glucose you ate recently and empty your muscle's stores so they are ready to accept new glucose the next time they see insulin. For those suffering from insulin resistance, the glucose use and glycogen depletion helps, however, working out consistently yields even more benefits. Your muscles need a source of energy and if you continue working, you will start to burn fat. As we know, stored fat only causes more problems for those with or developing insulin resistance and maintaining a healthy weight is very important for avoiding some of the vicious cycles of insulin resistance.

While we certainly don't consider our surroundings, our environment can have an impact on our likelihood of developing insulin resistance. Think about what foods are advertised around you on a daily basis. Sugary drinks and desserts are insanely popular in America and bacon and eggs for breakfast is being replaced by sugary cereals, juice, doughnuts and coffee with extra sugar and sugar filled fake chocolate, vanilla and caramel flavourings. At the grocery store you are bombarded with advertisements for high glycemic junk food. The checkout lane is filled with candy bars and store clerks get quite creative stacking cola crates into various eye-catching shapes. Added sugar is becoming an epidemic problem in western diets as the majority of the sugar we consume on average is pointless, processed, added sugar. Just look at a jar of popular tomato pasta sauce and you might be shocked to see that there is 7-10 grams of sugar (most of it added). Increased awareness is the only way to neutralize environmental factors. Look at nutrition labels, got to health food and natural food shops and improve your awareness on what kind of food you are buying.

In line with environment, stress plays a huge role in insulin resistance. Stress promotes the storage of more abdominal fat. More fat causes hormonal imbalances and the stress hormone, cortisol, creates all sorts of problems. A major problem is that stress makes our body think that we might need to fight or run soon and so our liver ramps up its production of glucose, causing a totally internal chain reaction of insulin resistance. Stress is blamed as an underlying cause for countless problems simply because it does cause a lot of problems. Our modern lives give us longer periods of sustained stress that or stone-age ancestors likely ever had to deal with. Stress causes so many more problems including systemic inflammation and immune suppression and again, every person has different bodily reactions to stress.

While we wish we could control all of these factors that lead to insulin resistance, one factor we cannot control is genetics. How we are created and come into this world and our ancestors have a huge, but varied effect on our lives. Obesity is one of the biggest correlating factors to insulin resistance and type 2 diabetes, a genetic predisposition for obesity can be difficult to overcome. Some surprising factors such as low birth weight have an impact on diabetes and insulin resistance risks. Finally, there are several flat out genes that correspond to a greater risk for type 2 diabetes and insulin resistance. Having these genetic factors can make it difficult to fight off insulin resistance, but it is far from a foregone conclusion.

* **Break the cycle**. We have talked endlessly about how insulin resistance creates a vicious cycle of escalating resistance and build-up of body fat, which causes further cyclical problems. If you are on the road to insulin resistance or diabetes then drastic action can yield strong benefits. As carbohydrates are the only significant trigger for insulin and thus insulin resistance, limiting your carbohydrates to 10% or less of your total calories can almost eliminate the progression of insulin resistance. Studies have shown that diabetics who cut to 10% or less carbs improve so much that many of them can eliminate many or all of their medications, including insulin shots. For those with insulin resistance the 10% or less diet can be used as a short term diet to break those cycles and hopefully a more moderate carbohydrate balance can be found for a more permanent diet.

* **Time your meals.** Late dinners and midnight snacks can be detrimental to insulin resistance. Insulin levels will normalize during the overnight fast between your evening meal and break-fast the following day, so increasing this fast by eating an early dinner and a later breakfast can help to fight insulin resistance. If you have snacks, try to make them high protein like nuts so that you feel fuller longer and are not tempted to eat more carbs.

* Balance your meals. We talked about how different foods are broken down and how they impact your blood sugar but it is important to know that all that food goes to the same place in order to break down. Eating a meal of pasta with sugary tomato sauce, garlic bread and a dessert of ice cream is carbs paired with carbs and more carbs causing a high and lasting blood sugar spike. Pairing quinoa or brown rice with fiber rich vegetables and lean meats provides a buffer that slows and lessens the impact of sugars. Ginger and cinnamon are great superfoods for blood sugar management but taking them during or immediately after a meal goes a long way in better managing blood sugar.

* Change shopping venues. Changing where you get your food can encourage better eating habits. Eating healthy is a lot easier if you only buy healthy foods. Try making your regular grocery stop a whole foods or natural food store where you can get less processed and packaged foods and more organic foods and healthy fruits and vegetables. Try going to your local farmer's market and pick up some fresh local produce. You might be amazed how skilled your local farmers are. It can be a fun and refreshing experience too.

* Lower your stress. Managing your stress can go a long way in reversing the road to insulin resistance. For some people, taking 5 minutes out of the day to relax does wonders. Yoga is an obvious stress reducer but even shutting the lights off and putting a cool compress over your eyes can slow or stop the stream of cortisol. Hopefully, you make the big life decisions like finding a career where you love going into work each morning. Little steps to reduce stress can count for a lot over the long term.

* Move! Yes exercise is extremely important and more exercise is almost always beneficial as most people rarely get to the point of overtraining. Even so, our lives and jobs can make it difficult to get in a full work out. This is not an excuse to sit around all day, but rather a challenge to find the parts of your day where you can be more active.

- Take the stairs to work.

- Adopt a standing desk; standing burns 50-100 calories more per hour than sitting and that's not counting any air squats or other fidgeting you might do.

- Try walking or biking to work. You can cover a lot more ground than you might realize, for those living and working in a city it might be faster to bike to work.

- Constantly think of ways to work yourself just a little bit more, park farther away, go for a nice walk outside, the possibilities are limitless.

* Pick the right foods. Knowing what to eat is very important as there are many surprising foods that can really speed up the development of insulin resistance. Here are some foods that are good at preventing or reversing insulin resistance.

- Green tea and coffee. The caffeine in these drinks actually promotes the release and burning of fat and can improve insulin sensitivity. In moderation, caffeine is actually quite healthy for those who can tolerate it. Aside from caffeine, coffee and tea have a host of other micronutrients and antioxidants important to leading a healthy life.

- Switch to unprocessed cooking oils like olive or coconut oil. These have a much greater ratio of healthy fats and lack the unhealthy man made fats found in processed or refined vegetable oils.

- Find organic omega 3 eggs. These eggs are not only protein rich and satisfyingly but they also have a higher ratio of omega 3 to saturated fat due to the chicken's diet and are all the better at controlling insulin resistance.

- Choose real, whole, unprocessed foods. The more processed a food is the greater chance that it has added sodium, fat and sugar. Our distant ancestors rarely had problems with insulin resistance or diabetes, so it's probably a good idea to follow their example when it comes to food choices.

Part 2: Recipes

This section is comprised of recipes designed to start you down the road to overcoming insulin resistance. These meals minimise refined sugar and carbohydrates to help you control blood sugar and fight insulin resistance.

Breakfast

Strawberry Banana Breakfast Bars (Low Sugar)

Prep time: 10 minutes
Cooking time: 45 minutes + 30 minutes cooling
Servings: 8 bars

Ingredients
1 ½ cups walnuts, chopped
1 ½ cups unsweetened coconut flakes
2 ripe bananas
1 tsp vanilla extract
½ tsp salt
Strawberry jam

Instructions
- Preheat the oven to 350°F/180°C.
- Line one loaf pan with parchment paper.
- In the bowl of a food processor, combine 1 cup walnuts and 1 cup coconut flakes. Pulse the mixture to break up into pieces. Add ripe bananas, vanilla extract and salt. Blend until the mixture is well combined.
- Place mixture in to a loaf pan, smoothen the top evenly with a rubber spatula and bake for about 25 minutes.

- Toast remaining coconut flakes in a skillet or frying pan over medium heat, stirring frequently. Transfer toasted coconut flakes in a small bowl and combine with remaining ½ cup walnuts.
- Spread a thin layer of strawberry jam over top of bars, then sprinkle the toasted coconut/walnut mixture on top, scattering evenly.
- Bake again for another 8-10 minutes or until golden brown.
- Remove the loaf pan out from the oven and set aside to cool.
- Slice the bars and refrigerate for about 30 minutes before serving.
- Store the remaining bar in the refrigerator.
- Best served chilled.

Carroty Coconutty Breakfast Loaf

Prep time: 15 minutes
Cooking time: 40 minutes
Servings: yields 1 loaf

Ingredients
¾ cup almond meal
1 tsp baking soda
½ tsp ground cinnamon
2 eggs
½ tsp vanilla extract
4 Tbsp coconut oil
½ cup ripe bananas, mashed
½ cup dates, pitted and chopped
½ cup carrots, grated
½ cup desiccated coconut
¼ cup hazelnuts or pistachios, chopped roughly
¼ cup cranberries

Instructions
- Preheat the oven to 350°F/180°C.
- Line a loaf pan or tin with parchment paper.
- Mix together almond meal, cinnamon and baking soda in a large bowl. Set aside.

- Whisk eggs in another bowl. Stir in coconut oil, vanilla and mashed bananas.
- In a large bowl, combine mashed banana mixture and almond meal mixture. Fold gently to combine.
- Add dates, grated carrots, desiccated coconut, chopped nuts and cranberries. Mix gently. There should be no lumps of dates sticking together.
- Transfer the batter into the loaf pan or tin and bake until cake tester comes out clean, about 40 minutes.

Apple Streusel Breakfast Muffins

Prep time: 15 minutes
Cooking time: 40 minutes
Servings: 12 muffins

Ingredients

2 cups green apples, cut into ½-inch pieces
3 Tbsp warm water
2 tsp cinnamon, divided
1 ½ Tbsp butter or coconut oil
9 eggs
3 Tbsp coconut milk
1 ½ Tbsp coconut flour
¼ tsp baking soda
Pinch of sea salt

Instructions

- Preheat oven to 350ºF/180ºC.
- Sauté the apples in a medium pan or skillet together with water and 1 ½ tsp cinnamon. Cook until apple consistency is like apple pie filling or chunky applesauce. Turn off the heat and let the mixture cool.

- Prepare the egg mixture by combining eggs, coconut milk, coconut flour, ½ tsp cinnamon, baking soda and salt in a medium-sized bowl. Whisk until well combined.
- Combine cooled apples and egg mixture. Reserve ¼ cup of the mixture for later use.
- Fill prepared muffin tins with the mixture, about ¼ cup each.
- Top each muffin with 1 tsp of the reserved mixture and bake for about 40 minutes.

Omelette Muffins

Prep time: 10 minutes
Cooking time: 20 minutes
Servings: 6 muffins

Ingredients

6 eggs
½ cup meat, cooked and cut into small pieces
½ cup vegetables of your choice, diced
¼ tsp salt
1/8 tsp ground black pepper
1/8 cup mayonnaise
1/8 cup water

Instructions

- Preheat oven to 350ºF/180ºC.
- Grease 6 muffin tins generously with butter or olive oil or line with paper muffin cups.
- Beat eggs in a large bow. Stir in remaining ingredients. Mix gently to combine.
- Spoon mixture into prepared muffin cups.
- Bake muffins until a knife or toothpick inserted into the center comes out clean, about 18 minutes.
- Serve muffin omelet hot or cold.

Zucchini and Carrot Breakfast Quiche

Prep time: 20 minutes
Cooking time: 45 minutes
Servings: 6

Ingredients
1 large zucchini, shredded and juice strained
2 large carrots, shredded
1 tsp rosemary-sage salt (optional)
12 eggs, beaten
1 Tbsp butter or coconut oil

Instructions
- Preheat oven to 375°F/190°C.
- In a large bowl, combine zucchini, carrots, Rosemary-Sage Salt, and eggs. Mix well and set aside.
- Brush a 9 inch x 13 inch baking dish generously with butter. Pour the egg mixture into the pan.
- Use a fork to create a swirled effect of circular pattern before baking.
- Bake quiche for until the edges are brown, about 45 minutes.
- It is normal for the quiche to puff up while baking and then deflate when removed from the oven.

Quiche of Asparagus, Mushroom and Spaghetti Squash

Prep time: 15 minutes
Cooking time: 1 hour 10 minutes
Servings: 4

Ingredients

1 spaghetti squash, halves and deseeded
13oz asparagus, trimmed and cut into 1-inch length
½ piece red onion, thinly sliced
1 cup mushrooms, sliced
2 garlic cloves, minced
5 eggs
½ cup coconut milk
1 tsp fresh rosemary, minced
Salt and ground black pepper to taste

Instructions

- Preheat the oven to 400°F/200°C.
- Place halved spaghetti squash face down on a baking sheet and bake for about 30 minutes. Remove from the oven and set aside to cool.
- Scrape the flesh of squash using a fork. Place squash in a bowl and set aside.

- Heat oil in a skillet over medium heat, then sauté onion and garlic until onion is soft.
- Stir in asparagus and mushrooms and sauté until asparagus is slightly tender but still crunchy. The moment it changes color, it is done.
- Meanwhile, in a bowl, whisk together eggs, coconut milk and rosemary. Season to taste with salt and ground black pepper.
- To make a crust for quiche, line a deep pie dish with cooked spaghetti squash. Press the spaghetti squash on the bottom and sides, pressing gently to make it even.
- Pour egg mixture over the squash. Spread mushrooms and asparagus on top of the egg mixture and bake in the oven for about 40 minutes or until set.

Tomato and Bacon Frittatas

Prep time: 10 minutes
Cooking time: 50 minutes
Servings: 4

Ingredients
4 ripe tomatoes, cut the tops off
4 eggs
4 slices bacon, cooked and diced
1 Tbsp ghee
Salt and pepper to taste
Fresh arugula for garnish

Instructions
- Preheat the oven to 425°F/200°C.
- Clean or scrape the inside of tomato using a spoon, to make a presentable tomato ramekin.
- Divide diced bacon on each tomato ramekin.
- Meanwhile, scramble the eggs and divide them evenly on each tomato ramekin. Alternatively, crack each egg on each tomato ramekin if you like poached egg.
- Divide ghee and top each tomato evenly and season each tomato with salt and ground black pepper.

- Place or arrange tomatoes evenly on a glass baking dish and bake until eggs are fully cooked, about 45 minutes.
- Place tomato frittatas on a serving platter with a garnish of fresh arugula.

Gruyere and Bacon Casserole

Prep time: 15 minutes
Cooking time: 55 minutes
Servings: 4-6

Ingredients
2 cups spaghetti squash strands, cooked
8oz organic nitrate-free bacon, cut into ½-inch pieces
1 yellow onion, chopped
4 eggs
4oz Gruyere cheese, shredded
1 tsp fine salt
Ground black pepper to taste

Instructions
- Preheat oven to 350°F/180°C.
- Grease an 8x8-inch glass baking dish generously with butter.
- Heat a large skillet over medium heat, then fry bacon pieces for about 5 minutes.
- Add chopped onion and sauté with the bacon for about 10 minutes or until onions are soft and the bacon is crispy.
- Transfer the sautéed mixture on a large mixing bowl. Add the cooked spaghetti squash and 3oz of shredded cheese. Season lightly with salt and ground black pepper. Mix gently.

- Spread mixture on the prepared baking dish and sprinkle with remaining cheese.
- Bake for about 40 minutes or until top is lightly golden and the center is set. Set aside for 15 minutes.
- Serve at room temperature.
- Store leftover casserole in a sealed container and refrigerate for up to 4 days.

Lunch

Greek Salad
Prep time: 10 minutes
Cooking time: 10 minutes
Servings: 8

Ingredients
3 cucumbers, seeded and sliced
1 ½ cups of Feta cheese, crumbled (made from goat's milk)
1 cup of black olives, pitted and sliced
3 cups of Roma tomatoes, diced
⅓ cup of diced, oil packed sun-dried tomatoes (drained, oil reserved)
½ red onion, sliced

Instructions
- In a large salad bowl, combine cucumbers, feta cheese, olives, Roma tomatoes, sun-dried tomatoes, 2 tablespoons reserved sun-dried tomato olive oil, and red onion. Toss together gently till combined.
- Chill just before serving.

Braised Beef Stew

Prep time: 15 minutes
Cooking time: 4 hours
Servings: 3-5

Ingredients
3 lb beef short ribs
3 Tbsp butter
3 stalks celery, diced
½ yellow onion, diced
2 carrots, diced
4 garlic cloves, minced
4 oz mushrooms, roughly chopped
A handful of sage, rosemary and thyme, chopped
4 cups chicken stock
2 cups roasted marinara sauce or tomato sauce
¼ cup apple cider vinegar
Salt and ground black pepper

Instructions
- Preheat the oven to 250°F/150°C.
- Melt the butter in a heavy bottomed ovenproof pot, over high heat.

- Sear the beef until golden brown crust is formed, then transfer beef to a large plate and set aside.
- To the same pot, add celery, onion, carrots, garlic and mushrooms and sauté until vegetables are tender but not overcooked.
- Stir in tomato sauce, vinegar and herbs.
- Place beef ribs back to the pot. Stir once. Place parchment paper on top of the pot to cover the stew then place inside the oven and cook for about 4 hours or until meat flakes easily with a fork.
- Remove the pot from the oven carefully, then gently separate the bones from the meat. Discard the bones.
- Let the meat cool down and use your fingers to pull apart the meat.
- Add flaked meat back to the pot and serve immediately.

Fire Roasted Tomato and Bacon Meatloaf

Prep time: 15 minutes
Cooking time: 60 minutes
Servings: 4

Ingredients
1 lb grass-fed ground beef
1 lb bacon, chopped
1 can (14oz) fire-roasted tomatoes
1 red onion, chopped
1 red bell pepper, chopped
3 garlic cloves, minced
2 eggs
1 cup almond flour
1 Tbsp oregano
½ Tbsp salt
Fresh ground black pepper to taste

Instructions
- Preheat the oven to 400°F/200°C.
- Combine chopped bacon and ground beef in a large mixing bowl, then add all ingredients and mix gently, using your hands. Mix well.

- Form mixture into loaf shape and place in a glass baking dish or pyrex dish or form into small meatballs and arrange in a baking sheet.
- Bake for about 1 hour or until the meat is cooked.
- Remove the meatloaf or meatballs out of the oven and set aside to cool for about 15 minutes.
- Sliced the meatloaf and serve with a drizzle of your favorite barbecue sauce.

Sausage Casserole

Prep time: 20 minutes
Cooking time: 45 minutes
Servings: 4-6

Ingredients

6 sausages
1 pint grape tomatoes
3 sweet potatoes
2 large bell pepper, chopped
1 red onion, chopped
2 garlic cloves, minced
Fresh thyme sprigs
Sea salt and fresh ground black pepper to taste

Instructions

- Preheat the oven to 400°F/200°C.
- In a large baking dish, spread grape tomatoes, sweet potatoes, red onion, bell pepper and minced garlic.
- Meanwhile heat the skillet and brown sausages on all sides, about 2 minutes per side.
- Scatter sausages over the vegetables, sprinkle thyme, some salt and ground black pepper.
- Bake sausage casserole for about 40 to 45 minutes.

Thai Pumpkin and Chicken Curry

Prep time: 10 minutes
Cooking time: 15-20 minutes
Servings: 4

Ingredients

1 Tbsp coconut oil
1 onion, thinly sliced
4 garlic cloves, minced
1 tsp salt
1 Tbsp Thai red curry paste
1 ⅓ cups coconut milk
⅓ cup pumpkin puree
1 ½ lbs boneless skinless chicken breast, cut into 1-inch cubes
2 tsp lime juice
¼ cup cilantro, chopped
3 Tbsp cashews, toasted

Instructions

- Heat the coconut oil in a large pan over medium heat, then sauté onion for about 5 minutes or until onion is soft.
- Sauté bell pepper, garlic and salt, stirring continuously for 1 minute.

- Stir in curry paste and cook for another 1 minute, stirring frequently.
- Pour in coconut milk, pumpkin puree and chicken, lower the heat and let the mixture simmer over low heat for about 12 minutes or until chicken is cooked.
- Stir in lime juice.
- Serve with a Garnish of fresh chopped cilantro and toasted cashews.

Fish Chowder with Plantain Croutons

Prep time: 10 minutes
Cooking time: 20 minutes
Servings: 4

Ingredients

For the Chowder
2 Tbsp coconut oil
1 tsp cumin seeds
1 tsp brown mustard seeds
1 thumb-size piece ginger, minced
1 yellow onion, diced
4 garlic cloves, minced
1 tsp curry powder
1 tsp garam masala
1 can coconut milk
2 lbs flaky white fish
Salt, to taste
2 Tbsp lime juice

For the Crou-tains
3 green plantains, diced
3 Tbsp coconut oil

salt

Instructions

- Melt coconut oil in a medium-sized soup pot over medium heat, then add cumin and mustard seed and sauté for about 2 minutes.
- Add ginger, garlic and onion and continue sautéing until onion is soft.
- Stir in curry and garam masala powder. Pour in can of coconut milk and stir the mixture to combine.
- Add fish. Stir the mixture gently once in a while until the fish are cooked. Fish is cooked when flesh flakes easily when prick with fork.
- Turn off heat, then stir in lime juice.
- Meanwhile, make the crou-tains; heat coconut oil in a large pan or skillet. Add diced plantain and fry until the plantains are cooked and the edges are crusty and golden. It takes around 15 minutes to achieve the nice crust.

Spicy Cocoa Beef Chili

Prep time: 20 minutes
Cooking time: 2-3 hours
Servings: 6-8

Ingredients

2 Tbsp coconut oil

2 cups onion, diced

4 garlic cloves, minced

2 lbs ground beef

1 tsp dried oregano

2 Tbsp chili powder

2 Tbsp ground cumin

1 ½ tsp unsweetened cocoa powder

1 tsp ground allspice

1 tsp salt

1 can (6oz) tomato paste

1 can (14.5oz) fire-roasted tomatoes

1 can (14.5oz) beef broth

1 cup water

Instructions

- Heat coconut oil in a large pot or heavy saucepan over medium heat.

- Add onion and sauté until soft and translucent, about 7 minutes.
- Add garlic and sauté until fragrant.
- Using your hands, crumble the ground beef into the pan. Mix well, stirring and pressing the lumps with a wooden spoon and cook until beef is no longer pink.
- Meanwhile, crush oregano into small bowl in between your fingers to release the flavor. Add chili powder, cocoa, cumin, allspice and salt. Mix well.
- Add this mixture to the pot. Stir.
- Stir in tomato paste and cook for about 2 minutes.
- Stir in fire-roasted tomatoes including its juice, beef broth and water. Stir gently. Bring mixture to a boil.
- Reduce the heat to low and let the mixture simmer over low heat for at least 2 hours.

Carrot Cardamom Soup

Prep time: 15 minutes
Cooking time: 45 minutes
Servings: 6

Ingredients

1 Tbsp coconut oil
2 large leeks (white and light green ends only), thinly sliced
Salt and ground black pepper, to taste
1 ½ lbs carrots, peeled and cut into ½-inch coins
¼ cup apple, diced
1 tsp fresh ginger, minced
½ tsp ground cardamom
4 cups chicken stock
½ cup coconut milk

Instructions

- Melt coconut oil in a medium pan over high heat, then add leeks and generous pinch of salt. Sauté leeks until soft, about 5 minutes.
- Stir in carrot, ginger, apple and cardamom. Sauté until fragrant.
- Pour in chicken stock and bring to a boil.

- Reduce the heat, cover the pan and let the soup simmer over low heat until carrots are soft, about 30 minutes. Stir in coconut milk.
- Pour the mixture into a food processor and process until smooth. Add salt and pepper as necessary.
- Serve in individual soup bowl and serve immediately.

Dinner

Sea Bass with Olive and Caper Sauce
Prep time: 15 minutes
Cooking time: 20 minutes
Servings: 4

Ingredients
10 whole green olives in brine
4 fillets (~ 5oz each) Fresh seabass
2 celery sticks, chopped
1 onion, finely chopped
Extra virgin olive oil
1 oz salted capers, well rinsed, drained and chopped
2 Tbsp of tomato puree
2 Tbsp of white wine vinegar
2 Tbsp of honey
½ cup fish stock
½ clove of garlic, minced
handful of fresh parsley, finely chopped

Instructions
- Use a sharp knife to make four cuts in each olive from end to end, and carefully remove each segments from the stone.

- Steam sea bass fillets over a pan of boiling water, covered, for about 12 minutes or until firm (cooking time depends on the thickness of the fish).
- Meanwhile, boil some water in a heavy saucepan and add the chopped celery and cook until the celery softens, about 1-2 minutes.
- Remove the celery from the boiling water, using a slotted spoon. Drain celery in a paper towel.
- To the same water, add the onion and cook for 1 minute, just to soften the onion.
- Remove the onion from the boiling water, using a slotted spoon. Drain onions in a paper towel.
- Heat the olive oil in a large skillet and sauté the pre-cooked celery and onions, stirring gently for a few minutes, then stir in the olives and capers and sauté for a few more minutes.
- Stir in tomato puree, vinegar, honey and fish stock. Cook over medium heat, stirring frequently until the liquid reduce and thickens slightly.
- Transfer the steamed fish fillets on a serving platter and pour the sauce over.
- Stir the chopped parsley and garlic together in bowl until well combined and sprinkle over the top. Serve.

Sicilian Meatballs

Prep time: 5 minutes
Cooking time: 20 minutes
Servings: 6-10 meatballs

Ingredients
1 lb ground grass fed beef or ground pork
½ tsp sea salt
¼ cup onion, minced
1 garlic clove, minced
1 ½ tsp Italian seasoning
¾ tsp dried oregano
1 egg, beaten
½ cup almond flour

Instructions
- Preheat the oven to 400°F/200°C.
- Prepare one baking sheet and line with parchment paper.
- In a large bowl, combine ground beef or pork, salt, minced onion and garlic, Italian seasoning, oregano, beaten egg and almond flour. Mix well.
- Form mixture into meatballs. Make small or big ones, just adjust the baking time.

- Arrange meatballs in a baking sheet and bake for about 20 minutes or until the meatballs are cooked.

Chicken, Coconut and Lime Soup

Prep time: 20 minutes
Cooking time: 20 minutes
Servings: 4

Ingredients
2 lbs cooked chicken, cut into bite-sized pieces
15oz coconut milk
3 cups chicken broth
¼ cup lime juice
3 medium carrots, shredded
1 cup broccoli, shredded
1 cup rutabaga, shredded
2 tsp Thai seasoning
1 lime, cut into wedges
Salt and ground black pepper to taste

Thai Seasoning
½ tsp curry powder
¼ tsp cinnamon
¼ tsp ginger
¼ tsp chili powder
¼ tsp paprika
¼ tsp salt

Instructions

- In a large soup pot, combine chicken broth, lime juice, coconut milk, shredded vegetables, Thai seasoning and chicken. Season to taste with salt and ground black pepper.
- Bring soup to a boil. Lower the heat and let the soup simmer over low heat, covered, until vegetables are slightly tender, about 15 minutes.
- Serve warm with lime wedges.

Slow Cooked Chicken Coriander Enchilada Soup

Prep time: 15 minutes
Cooking time: 8 hours+
Servings: 4-6

Ingredients

1 ½ lbs boneless skinless chicken breast

1 yellow onion, diced

1 red bell pepper, sliced into thin strips

1 jalapeno, diced

2 garlic cloves, minced

1 can (15oz) diced tomatoes

2 cups chicken stock

1 Tbsp chili powder

1 Tbsp cumin

1 tsp dried oregano

½ tsp paprika

Salt and ground black pepper, to taste

2 Tbsp fresh cilantro, chopped

1 avocado, pitted and sliced

Instructions

- Place chicken on the bottom of a slow cooker.

- On top of the chicken, scatter diced onion, bell pepper, jalapeno and garlic.
- Pour diced tomatoes and chicken stock on top, then sprinkle with chili powder, cumin, oregano and paprika. Season lightly with salt and ground black pepper.
- Cover the slow cooker and cook the mixture on lowest settings for 8 hours.
- When cooked, shred chicken with a fork and place on a serving platter with a garnish of chopped fresh cilantro and sliced avocado.

Pork, Bacon and Apple Meatloaf

Prep time: 20 minutes
Cooking time: 1 hour
Servings: 4

Ingredients
1 ½ lb ground pork
1 ½ cup apples, peeled and grated
1 small onion, minced
1 Tbsp chili powder
1 tsp ground cinnamon
1 tsp dry mustard
7 slices bacon
Applesauce
Salt and fresh ground black pepper to taste

Instructions
- Preheat the oven to 350°F/180°C.
- Line a baking sheet with parchment paper.
- Combine ground pork, apples, onion, chili powder and cinnamon. Season to taste with salt and fresh ground black pepper.

- Shape mixture into loaf and place on a baking sheet. Lay bacon slices on top of the loaf, tucking the bacon underneath to tighten it.
- Bake loaf for about 1 hour.
- Preheat the broiler and broil meatloaf for about 3 minutes or until the bacon is crispy.
- Slice the meatloaf and serve with apple sauce.

Nicoise Salad

Prep time: 10 minutes
Cooking time: 20 minutes
Servings: 4

Ingredients
12-15 baby potatoes, unpeeled and thickly sliced
2 Tbsp of olive oil
4 eggs
2 Tbsp of capers, rinsed
1.8oz Sun Blush or sun dried tomatoes in oil, finely chopped
½ red onion, thinly sliced
3.5oz baby spinach
2 x cans (~15oz each) yellow fin tuna steak in spring water, drained

Instructions
- Preheat oven to 200ºC/fan 180ºC/gas 6.
- Season the potatoes with 2 tsp oil and salt+pepper.
- Arrange potatoes on a large baking pan and roast, stirring halfway until crisp and golden brown, about 20 minutes.
- Meanwhile, boil the eggs depending on how you liked them cooked.
- Submerge eggs into a bowl of cold water, then peel away the shells and cut each egg in half.

- Whisk the remaining oil in a salad bowl, together with red wine vinegar, capers and chopped tomatoes.
- Stir in the onions, spinach, tuna and potatoes. Toss everything together.
- Garnish salad with boiled eggs and serve immediately.

Beef Meatballs

Prep time: 5 minutes
Cooking time: 25 minutes
Servings: 12-16 meatballs

Ingredients
2 lbs grass-fed ground beef
4 eggs
2 cups carrots, shredded
½ onion, chopped
1 cup almond meal
1 tsp dried oregano
1 tsp dried basil
1 tsp dried Italian seasoning
1 tsp garlic powder
1 tsp salt
½ tsp ground pepper

Instructions
- Preheat the oven to 350°F/180°C.
- Line a baking sheet with parchment paper or grease with a little oil.

- In a large bowl, combine all ingredients and mix well using your hands. Form mixture into meatballs and bake for about 25 minutes or until the meatballs are cooked.

Malaysian Pork Curry

Prep time: 20 minutes
Cooking time: 45 minutes
Servings: 6-8

Ingredients
3 Tbsp curry paste (red, green, Panang or Massaman)
1 can coconut milk
2 tsp garlic, minced
2 onions, sliced
3 cups (750ml) chicken broth
1 green bell pepper, chopped
1 red bell pepper, chopped
1 yellow squash, cut into chunks
1 lb (450gram) okra, cut each pieces in half crosswise
3 kaffir lime leaves
1 lb (450gram) smoked pork butt, shredded or chopped
1 lb (450gram) andouille sausage, sliced
½ cup (12gram) Thai basil leaves
10 Thai peppers

Instructions
- Heat the curry paste in a large pan or Dutch oven until the color darkens and aromatic.

- Stir in ½ can of coconut milk and combine well with the curry paste. Stir until smooth.
- Stir in garlic and onion and the remaining coconut milk. Cook until onion is soft.
- Add chicken broth, squash, okra, peppers and kaffir lime leaves and let the mixture simmer for about 10 minutes.
- Cut or shred pork into large pieces and add to pot. Add basil and andouille sausage.
- Chop ½ of Thai pepper and add them to the mixture if you want it hot.
- Cook over low heat until okra is tender, about 25 minutes.
- Serve curry with cauliflower rice and a garnish of remaining Thai pepper.

Bacon Cinnamon Rolls with Icing

Prep time: 10 minutes
Cooking time: 20 minutes
Servings: 2

For the rolls
6 Slices unsmoked back bacon
2 Large eggs
5 Tbsp Clarified butter or ghee
3 Tbsp Raw natural honey
2.5 cups Almond flour
0.5 tsp Sea salt
0.5 tsp Baking soda
3 tsp Cinnamon
0.5 tsp Vanilla extract

For the icing
4 Tbsp Coconut butter
4 Tbsp Coconut milk

- Preheat the oven to 350ºF/180ºC and add the bacon slices to cook for a few minutes. They don't need to be crispy, just cooked through.

- Meanwhile, begin making the dough by cracking the eggs into a mixing bowl and adding 4 Tbsp of butter and 1 Tbsp of the honey. Mix until well combined.

- Add the almond flour, baking soda and salt to the bowl and mix again to combine until you have dough like consistency.

- Turn out the dough onto a large piece of baking parchment on top of a baking tray and place another piece of baking parchment on top of the dough. Use a rolling pin or bottle to roll the dough into a flat rectangle in the baking tray.

- Combine the remaining Tbsp of butter and 2 Tbsp honey into a small bowl and mix with a fork, then spread the mixture evenly over the rectangle of dough.

- Remove the cooked bacon from the oven and place evenly across the rectangle of dough. Use the parchment paper to roll the sheet from the edges into a circular roll.

- Use a sharp knife the cut the roll crossways into 6 pieces and bake in the oven for 20 minutes.

- Meanwhile, make the icing by combining the coconut milk and coconut butter in small bowl. Remove the rolls from the oven and drizzle with the icing to serve.

Honey-Caramelized Figs with Yogurt

Prep time: 10 minutes

Cooking time: 10 minutes

Servings: 4

Ingredients

1 Tbsp of honey, plus more for drizzling

8 ounce of fresh figs, halved

2 cups of plain Greek yogurt

Pinch of ground cinnamon

¼ cup of pistachios, chopped

Instructions

- Pour honey in a non-stick skillet and heat over low-heat.

- Add figs, cut side down and cook until caramelizes, about 5 minutes.

- Serve caramelized figs over yogurt with a sprinkling of cinnamon and top with pistachios.

- Drizzle with honey before serving.

Quick and Easy Pancakes with Fruit

Prep time: 10 minutes

Cooking time: 10 minutes

Servings: 4

Ingredients

1½ large ripe bananas

2 eggs

½ tsp. vanilla extract

¼ tsp. ground cinnamon

⅛ tsp. baking powder

Your choice of fresh fruits – apple, pear, blueberries etc.

Yoghurt or Maple syrup to serve (optional)

Instructions

- Crack the eggs into a large bowl and whisk

- In another bowl, mash up the bananas with a potato masher or a fork.

- Add the egg, baking powder, vanilla extract and the cinnamon to the mashed bananas and stir until well combined.

- Melt a little butter in a skillet placed over a medium-low heat/

- Pour about 2 tablespoons of the batter at a time onto the skillet and cook until the bottom appears set (1 to 2 minutes). Flip with a spatula and cook another minute.

- Serve immediately, topped with fresh fruit and maple syrup.

Apple Cobbler
Prep time: 10 minutes
Cooking time: 15-20 minutes
Servings: 4

Ingredients
3 Tbsp of butter
1 tsp of lemon juice
2 lbs apples, peeled, cored and chopped
1/3 cup of apple juice concentrates
¼ cup of raisins
½ tsp of vanilla extract
½ tsp of ground cinnamon
¼ tsp of ground ginger
¼ tsp of grated nutmeg

Topping
3 Tbsp of tapioca flour
1 Tbsp of coconut flour
½ stick (2oz) cold butter, cut into small cubes
1 Tbsp of apple juice concentrates

Instructions
- Preheat the broiler and place oven rack in the middle layer of the oven.

- Melt the butter in a medium cast iron skillet over medium-high heat and add in the lemon juice, apples, apple concentrate, raisins, vanilla, cinnamon, ginger and nutmeg. Stir to combine.
- Continue cooking until the apple juice concentrate has reduced and thickens, about 6 minutes. Turn off heat.
- Meanwhile, prepare the topping by combining tapioca and coconut flour.
- Add the butter into the flour and rub the mixture using your hands to create crumbs. Stir in apple juice slowly.
- Sprinkle this topping mixture on top of cooked apples and broil in the oven until top is golden brown, about 5 to 6 minutes.

Sticky Date Muffin Cupcakes

Prep time: 15 minutes

Cooking time: 25 minutes

Servings: 5

Ingredients

<u>For the muffins</u>

Butter for greasing

10 Tbsp water

12 dates

1½ ripe banana, peeled and roughly chopped

3 Tbsp coconut flour

1 Tbsp vanilla extract

2 eggs

½ tsp baking powder

<u>For the ganache</u>

5-6 dates, chopped

½ of orange, juice only

3 tbsp almond milk (coconut milk or water can also be used)

1 tsp vanilla extract or essence

1 tsp honey

Fresh raspberries or cherries for garnish

Instructions

- Preheat oven to 185°C/365 °F.

- Grease muffin tins with the butter and set aside.

- Heat the dates and water in a small saucepan over low heat until the dates disintegrate and thicken. Use a fork to mash them together and set aside.
- Combine the coconut flour, egg, banana, vanilla extract and baking powder in a food processor and process until well mixed and bubbly.
- Add the dates to the banana mixture and stir. Evenly distribute the mixture into the ramekins, then cook in the oven for 20 minutes.
- While the muffins are in the oven, place the sticky date ganache ingredients in a small saucepan over a low heat and cook until the dates break down and thicken, about 3-4 minutes.
- Mash with a fork and whisk until thickened. Set aside.
- Allow the muffins to rest for 5 minutes before removing them to a serving plate. Scoop a dollop of sticky date ganache paste on top and garnish with a few raspberries or cherries.

References

Overcoming Insulin Resistance

by Antony Jason Willfour

---

[1] http://www.diabetes.org/diabetes-basics/statistics/
[2] http://en.wikipedia.org/wiki/Insulin_resistance#Signs_and_symptoms
[3] http://www.aafp.org/afp/1998/1015/p1355.html
[4] http://www.mayoclinic.org/diseases-conditions/type-2-diabetes/basics/definition/con-20031902

CPSIA information can be obtained
at www.ICGtesting.com
Printed in the USA
LVHW011633230621
690870LV00013BB/816